What Happens Next?

DEALING WITH LIFE CHANGES

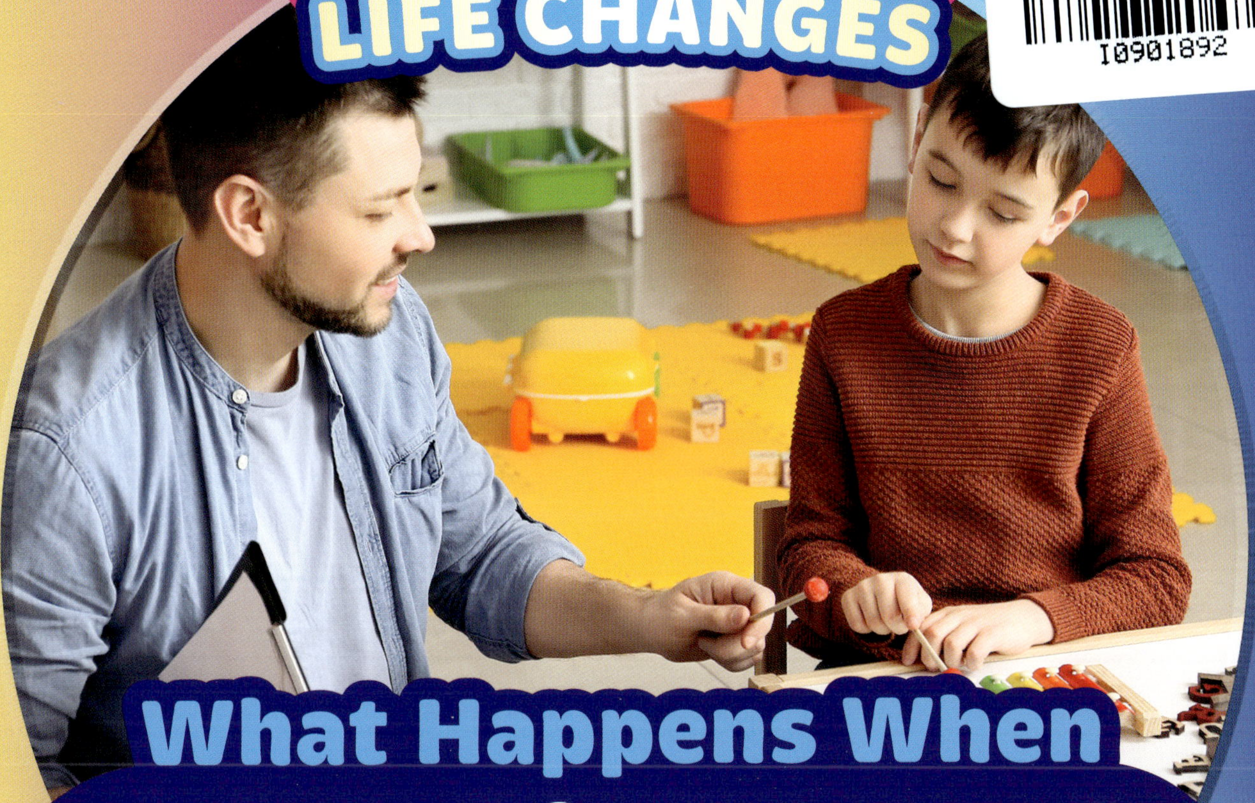

What Happens When I Am Diagnosed with Autism?

Danielle Haynes

PowerKiDS press

Published in 2025 by The Rosen Publishing Group, Inc.
2544 Clinton Street, Buffalo, NY 14224

First Edition

Editor: Theresa Emminizer
Book Design: Leslie Taylor

Photo Credits: Cover Pixel-Shot/Shutterstock.com; p. 5 Ground Picture/Shutterstock.com; p. 7 Ground Picture/Shutterstock.com; p. 9 Sergey Novikov/Shutterstock.com; p. 11 Kawin Ounprasertsuk/Shutterstock.com; p. 13 stockpexel/Shutterstock.com; p. 15 Peakstock/Shutterstock.com; p. 17 Prostock-studio/Shutterstock.com; p. 19 Tatiana Buzmakova/Shutterstock.com; p. 21 Dmytro Zinkevych/Shutterstock.com.

Cataloging-in-Publication Data

Names: Haynes, Danielle.
Title: What happens when I am diagnosed with autism? / Danielle Haynes.
Description: Buffalo, NY : PowerKids Press, 2025. | Series: What happens next? dealing with life changes| Includes glossary and index.
Identifiers: ISBN 9781725327054 (pbk.) | ISBN 9781725327078 (library bound) | ISBN 9781725327085 (ebook)
Subjects: LCSH: Autism–Juvenile literature. | Autism–Diagnosis–Juvenile literature. | Autism–Treatment–Juvenile literature.
Classification: LCC RC553.A88 H39 2025 | DDC 616.85'882–dc23

Manufactured in the United States of America

CPSIA Compliance Information: Batch #CSPK25. For Further Information contact Rosen Publishing at 1-800-237-9932.

CONTENTS

What Now?

A doctor just **diagnosed** you with autism. Your mind is probably filled with lots of questions and worries. What is autism? What does it mean for my **future**? Can I still go to school with my friends? Should I be scared?

There's a lot to learn about this disorder. You might need to find different ways to learn and live. But many people view autism spectrum disorder as a superpower! You have a one-of-a-kind way of viewing the world.

Your Point of View

No one's really sure what causes autism. It often runs in families, so if one of your parents has it, you might too. Being born premature, or early, may also increase your risk.

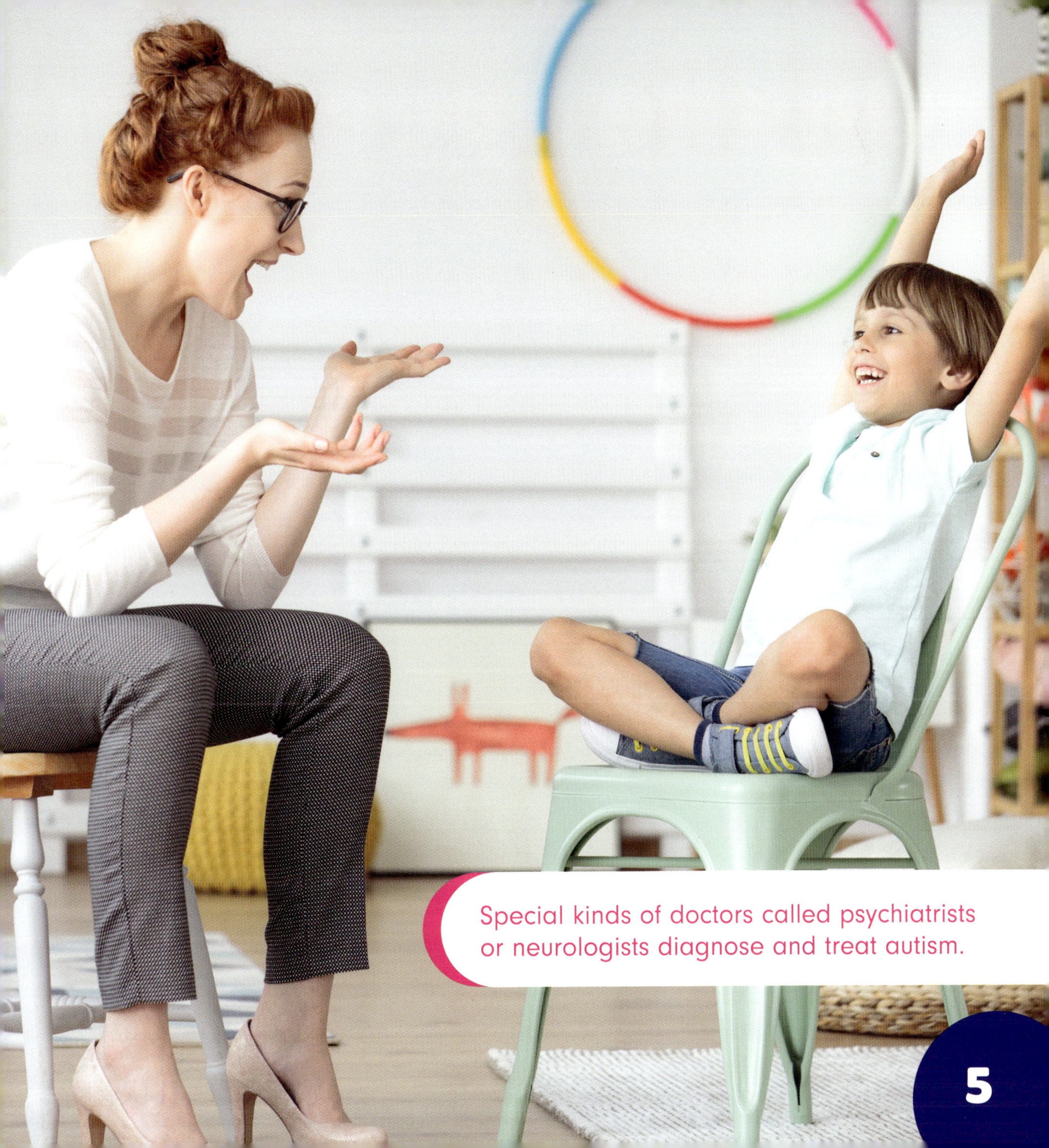

Special kinds of doctors called psychiatrists or neurologists diagnose and treat autism.

On the Spectrum

The full name for autism is autism spectrum disorder (ASD). "Spectrum" is another word for range. People with autism can have a range of many different symptoms, or signs.

Signs of autism may include troubles with:

- **communication**
- social skills
- loud noises
- touch
- **mental** health
- sleeping
- learning
- other health issues

Some people have stronger symptoms than other people. One person may have learned to speak late in life. Another may not speak at all. Like most things in life, everyone's a little different.

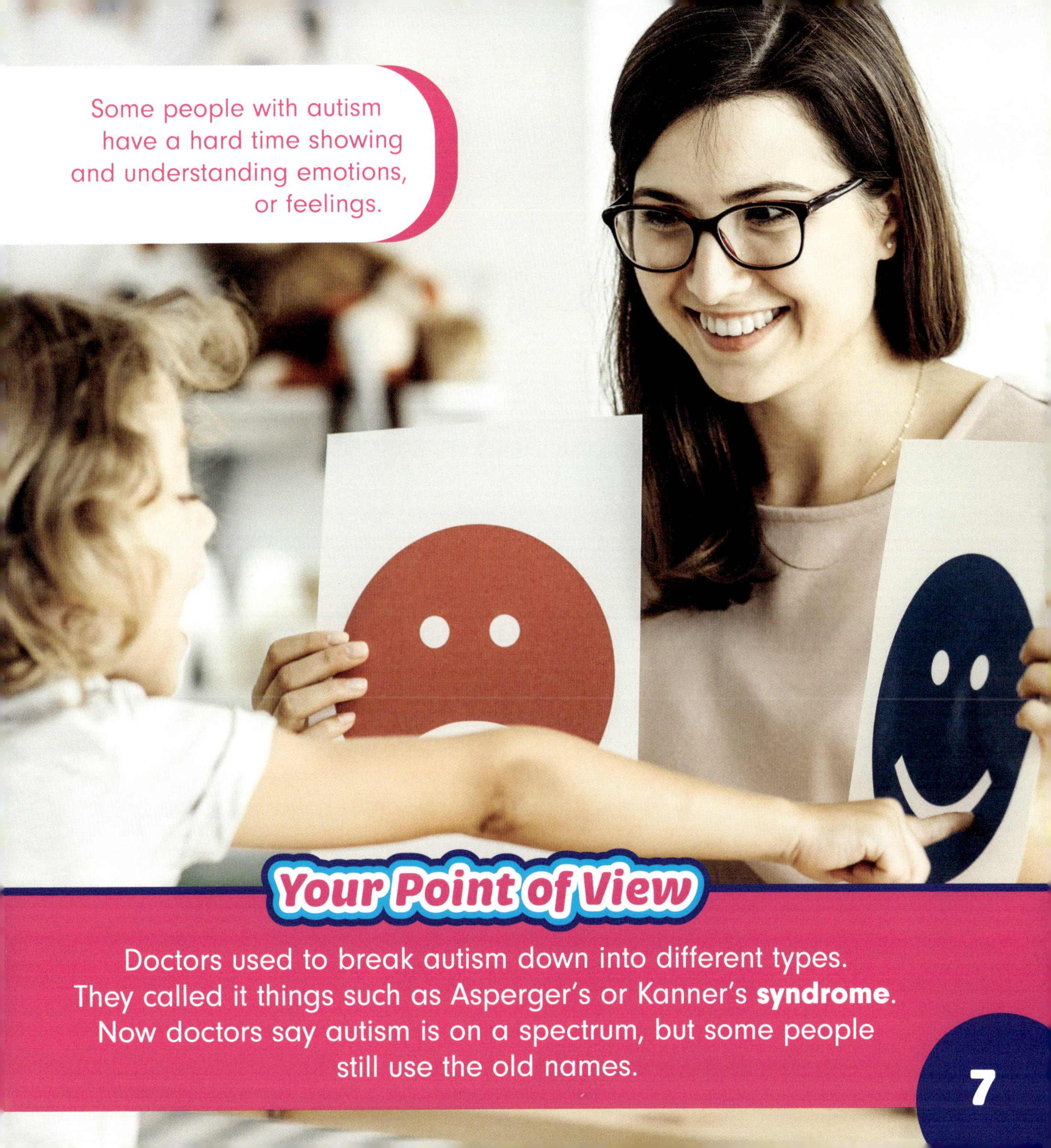

Some people with autism have a hard time showing and understanding emotions, or feelings.

Your Point of View

Doctors used to break autism down into different types. They called it things such as Asperger's or Kanner's **syndrome**. Now doctors say autism is on a spectrum, but some people still use the old names.

Neurodiversity

Doctors may say people with autism are neurodivergent. "Neuro" means something that deals with the brain" and "divergent" means different. People who are neurodiverse have brains that work differently than average people. Average people are called neurotypical.

Other neurodivergent conditions include dyslexia (difficulty reading), attention-deficit hyperactivity disorder (ADHD), and Down syndrome. Each of these conditions can cause issues with learning or in social settings. Being neurodivergent doesn't mean you're sick or your brain is broken. It just means you have a special way of learning!

Some people have more than one neurodivergent condition.

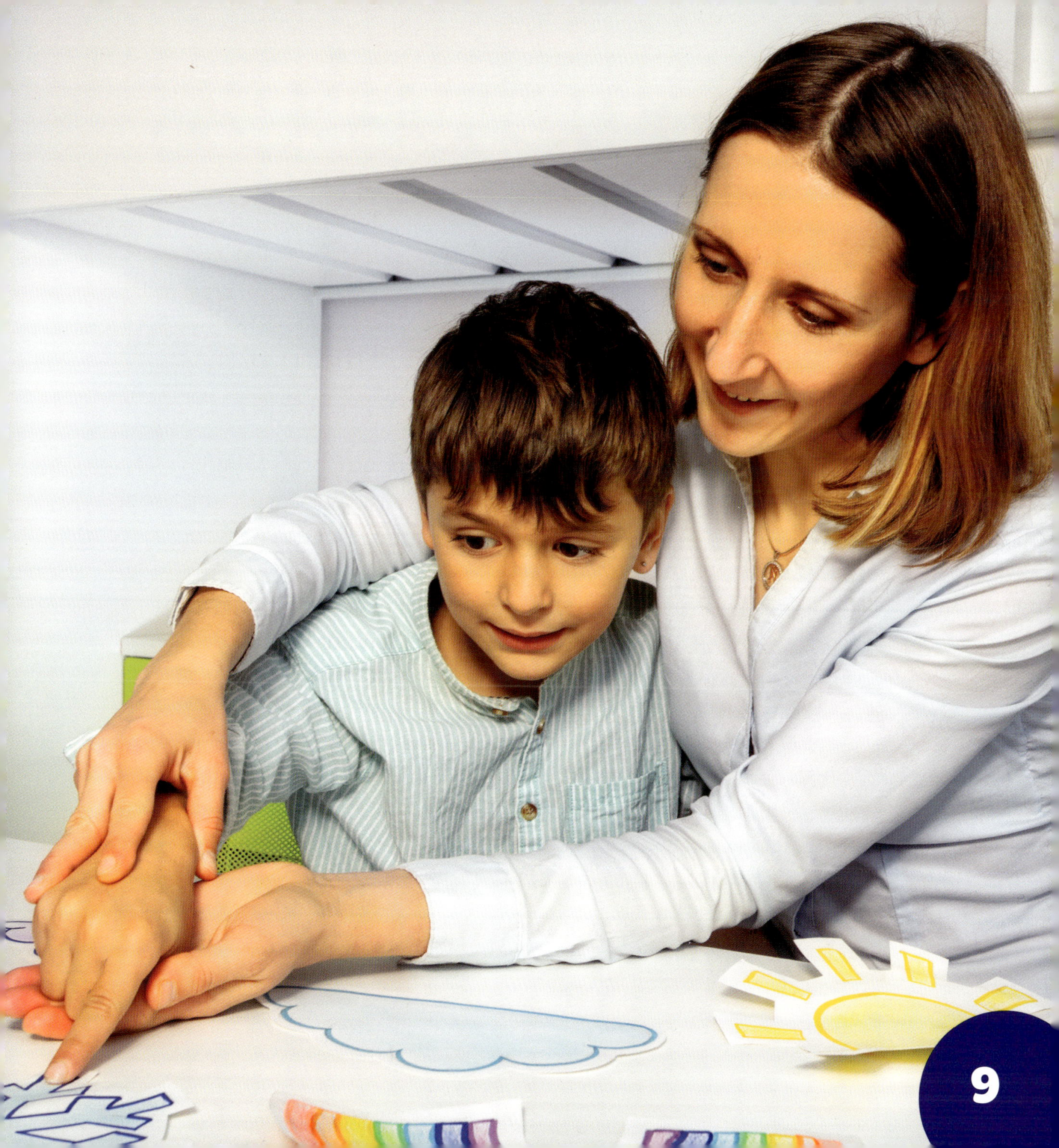

Superpowers!

Some of the signs of autism and neurodiversity may make it seem like you have superpowers! Some people with autism may find it easier to focus, or pay attention to, tasks than other people. Some are very creative or have strong memories. Others have a special talent in coming up with new ways of doing things.

Because of this, you may find that many people with autism have surprising gifts. You might be really good at playing musical instruments or drawing even if you've never had lessons!

Your Point of View

Some people with autism also have savant syndrome. This is a rare condition that makes someone unusually talented at different skills, such as playing piano or memorizing facts.

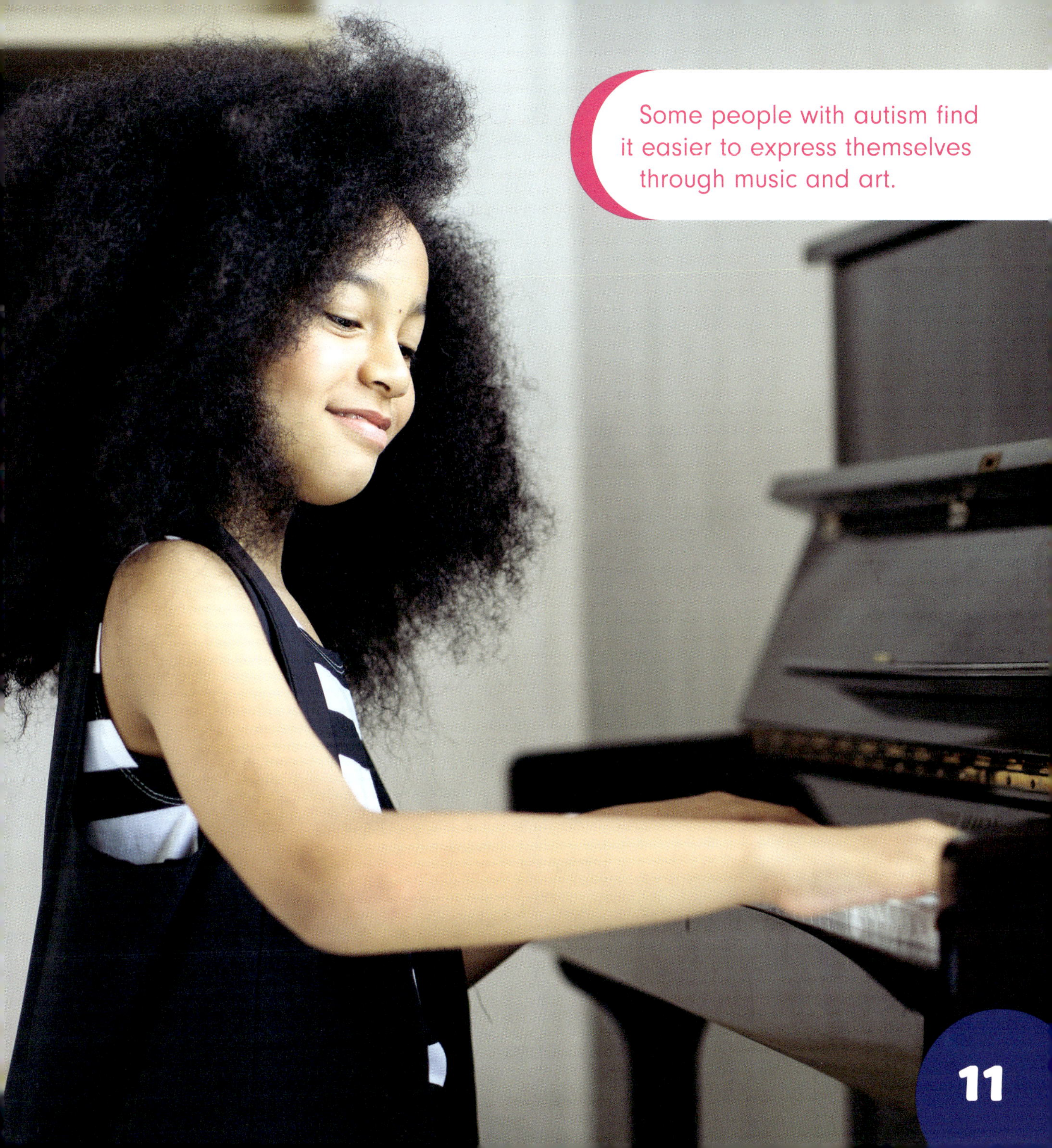

Some people with autism find it easier to express themselves through music and art.

Invisible Difference

Autism is thought to be an invisible difference. That means people can't immediately tell you have autism when they look at you. But just because you may not look like you have this difference doesn't mean you don't need help.

Because autism can't always be seen, it might be hard for friends, family, and strangers to understand why a person with autism might behave in a certain way. They might not know that you don't like hugs or that movie theaters are too loud for you.

Anyone can have an invisible difference or disorder, so it's important to be open minded and understanding.

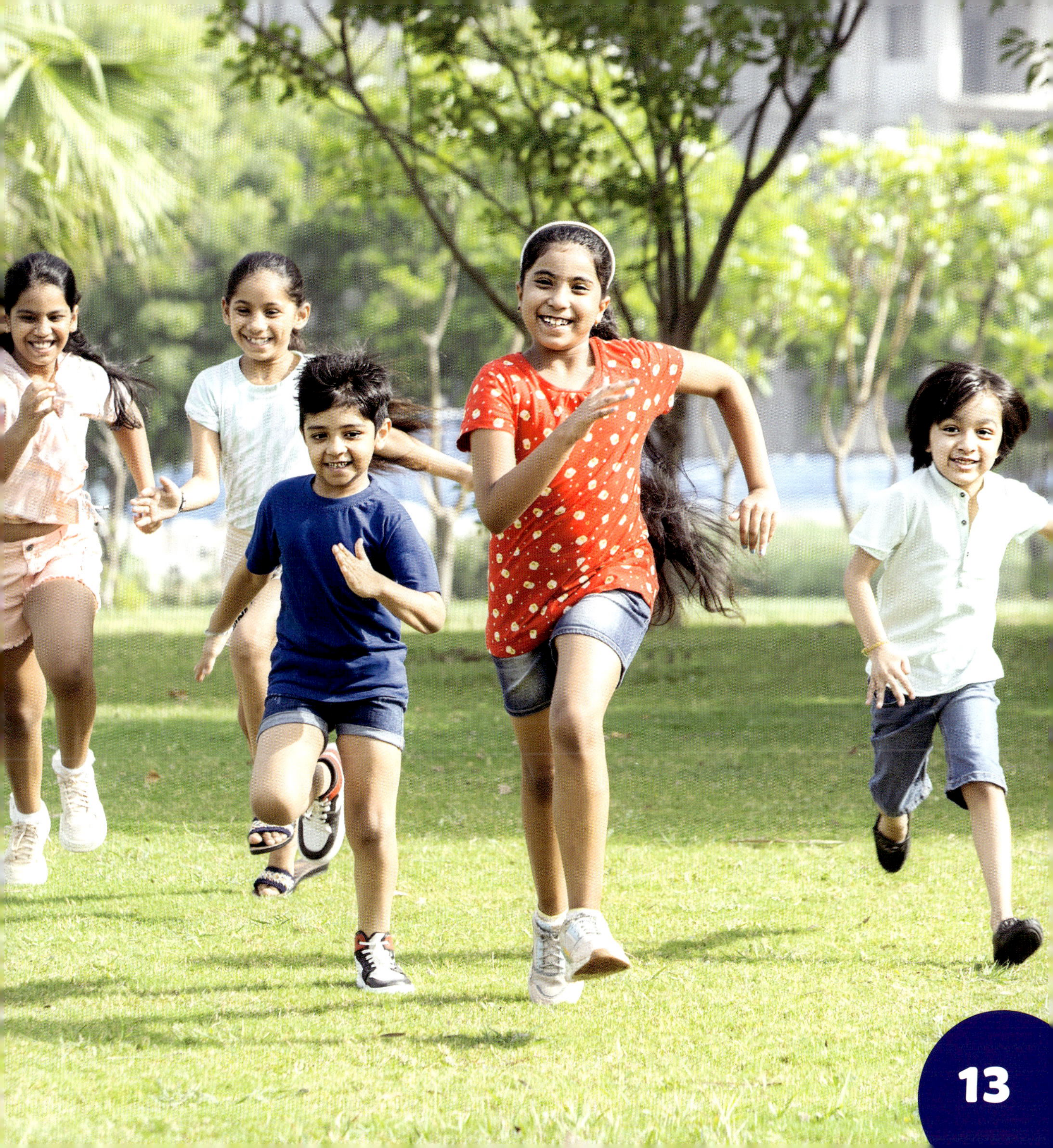

Getting Treatment

Now that you know you have autism, what do you do? Doctors and teachers have lots of ways to help you deal with your diagnosis. Different **treatments** can help different symptoms.

You might have to visit doctors or **therapists** regularly. Sometimes you might have to take medicine. You might need to eat or avoid certain foods. Your school may set up programs to match your learning style. No matter what, you have the right to get the best treatment for your unique, or one-of-a-kind, case!

Your Point of View

Some people with autism take medication to help symptoms. Some of these medicines might help you feel less **anxious**, sad, or angry. They may help you pay attention better in class.

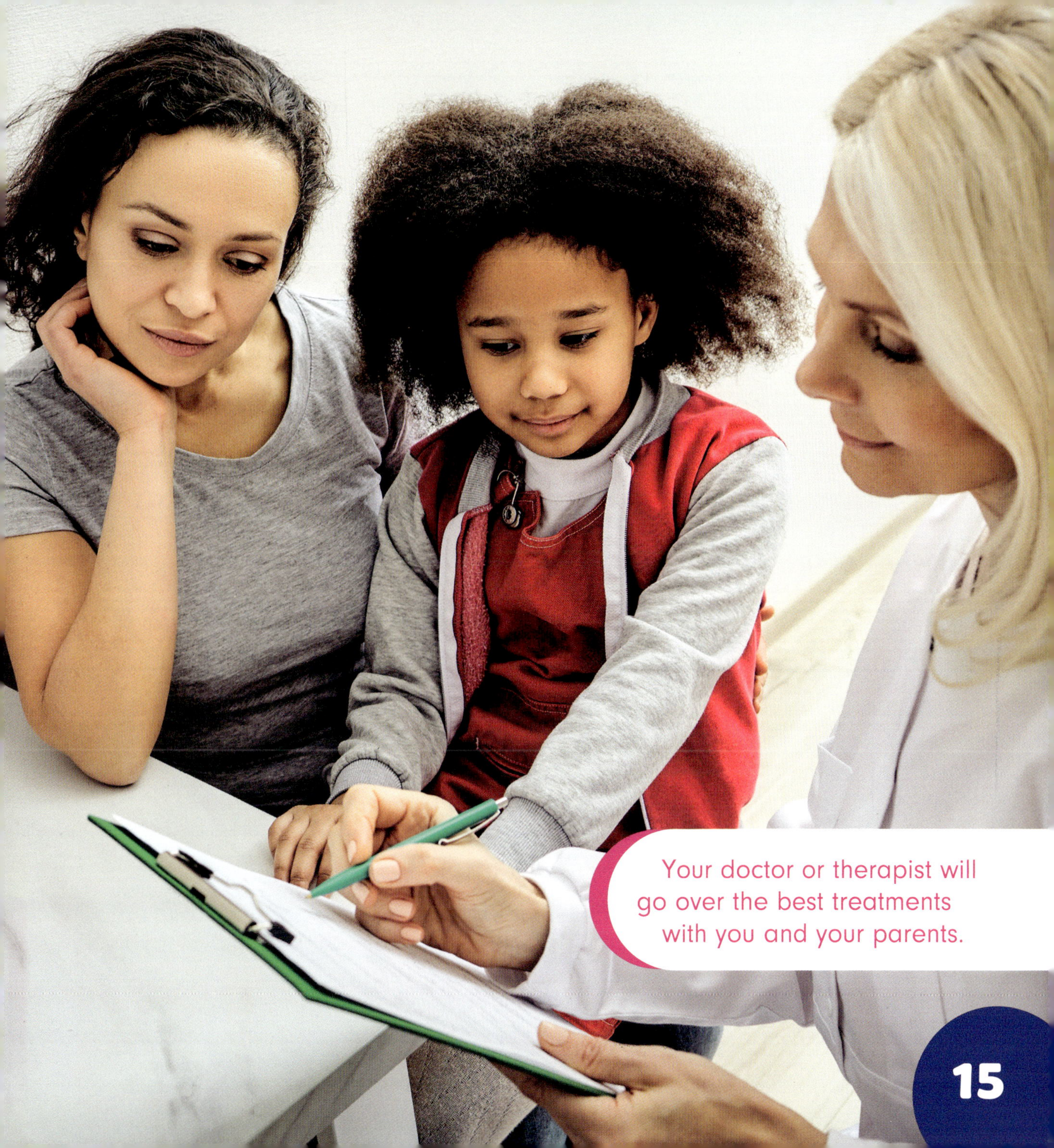

Your doctor or therapist will go over the best treatments with you and your parents.

Many people with autism get some kind of therapy. There are many kinds of therapy, not just the kind that deals with your emotions.

Physical therapy is helpful for people who need to work on grabbing things with their hands or keeping their balance.

Speech-language therapy helps people who have trouble speaking.

Behavioral management therapy stops unwanted actions and strengthens positive actions.

Some autistic people don't eat well because many foods taste or feel bad to them. Nutritional therapy helps with that.

Some people with autism are nonverbal, meaning they don't speak. Speech therapy helps them learn how to shape sounds with their mouth.

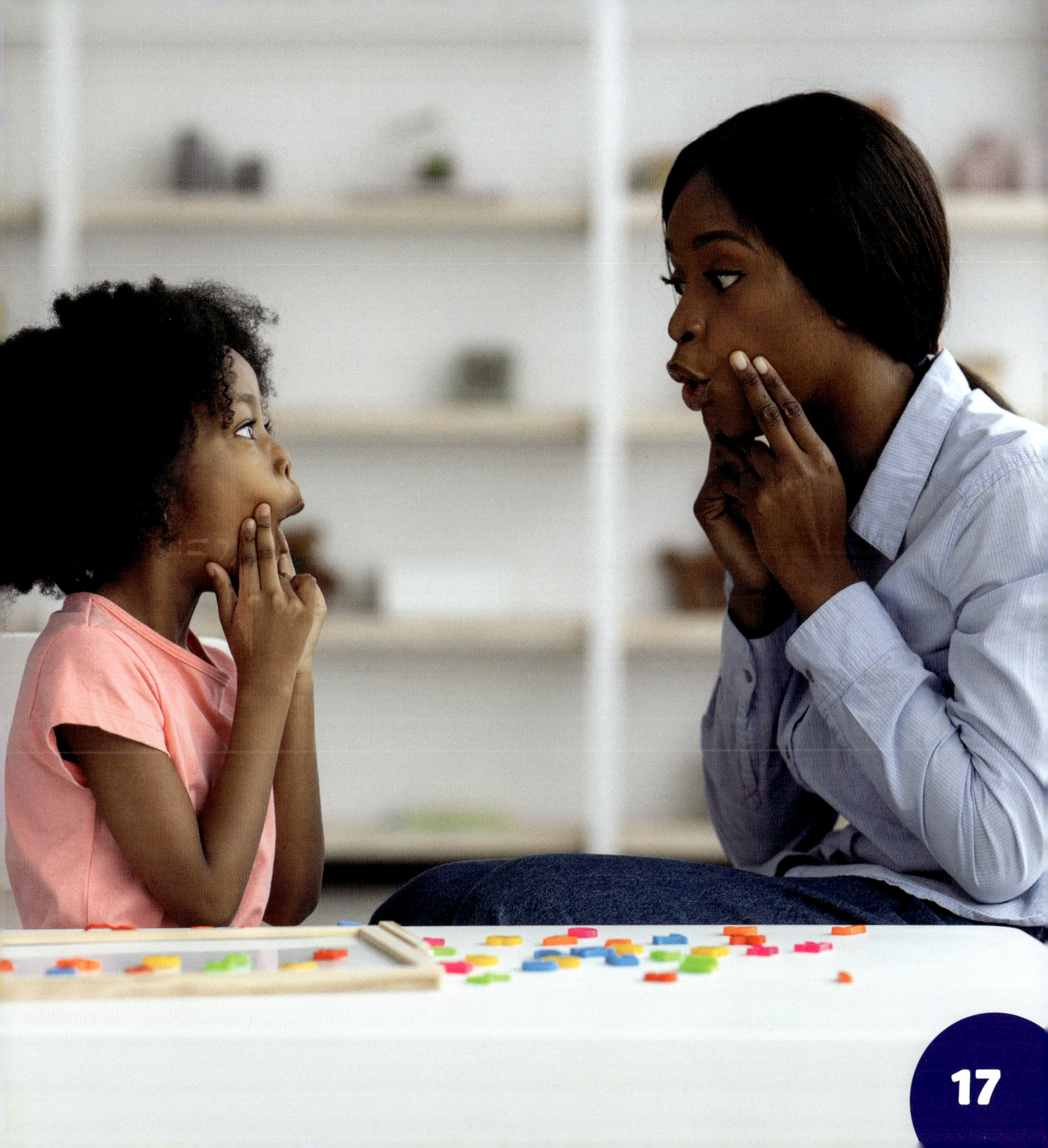

Autism and School

Teachers can play an important part in an autistic person's life. Sometimes they're the first person to notice signs of autism. They might bring up these symptoms to your guardians, or grown-ups at home. They might let a school **counselor** know.

And they'll most likely help you after your diagnosis. Since autism often **affects** how a person learns, it's important you get accommodations in your studies. Accommodations are changes made in class to help you learn.

Your Point of View

Some examples of accommodations are fidget toys or headphones that block loud noises. Teachers might also give students more time for tests.

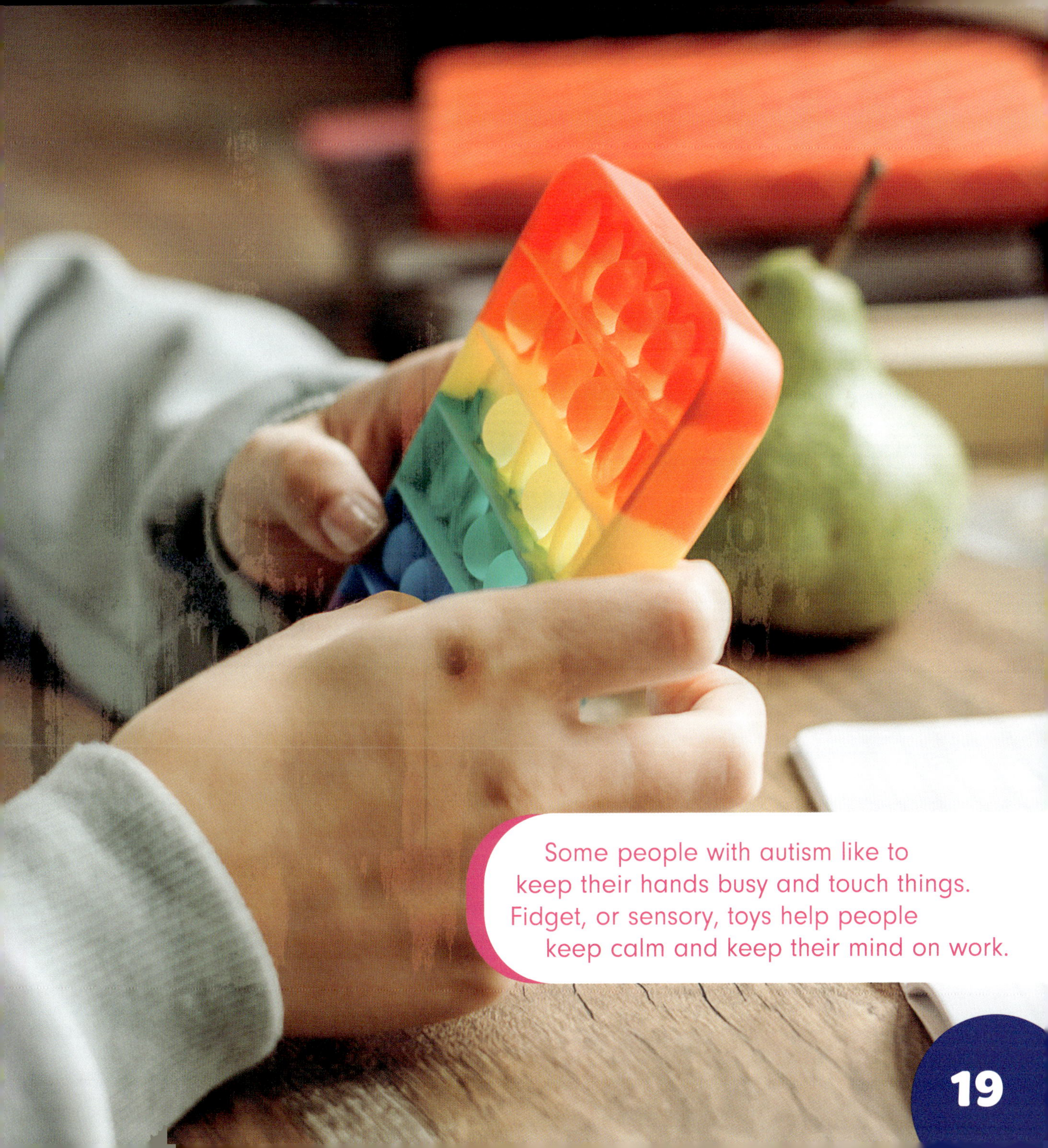

Some people with autism like to keep their hands busy and touch things. Fidget, or sensory, toys help people keep calm and keep their mind on work.

Bright Future

It can be scary visiting doctors and learning you have a disorder. That's totally normal! But after you learn a little bit more about autism, you can start to worry less and look to your future.

There are many options for help, including therapy, medication, and accommodations at school. You and your teachers, doctors, and family can team up to make autism work for you, not against you. You can make it your superpower!

Your Point of View

Your school can set up something called an Individualized Education Program (IEP). This plan will help your teachers make sure you have what you need to succeed as a student with autism.

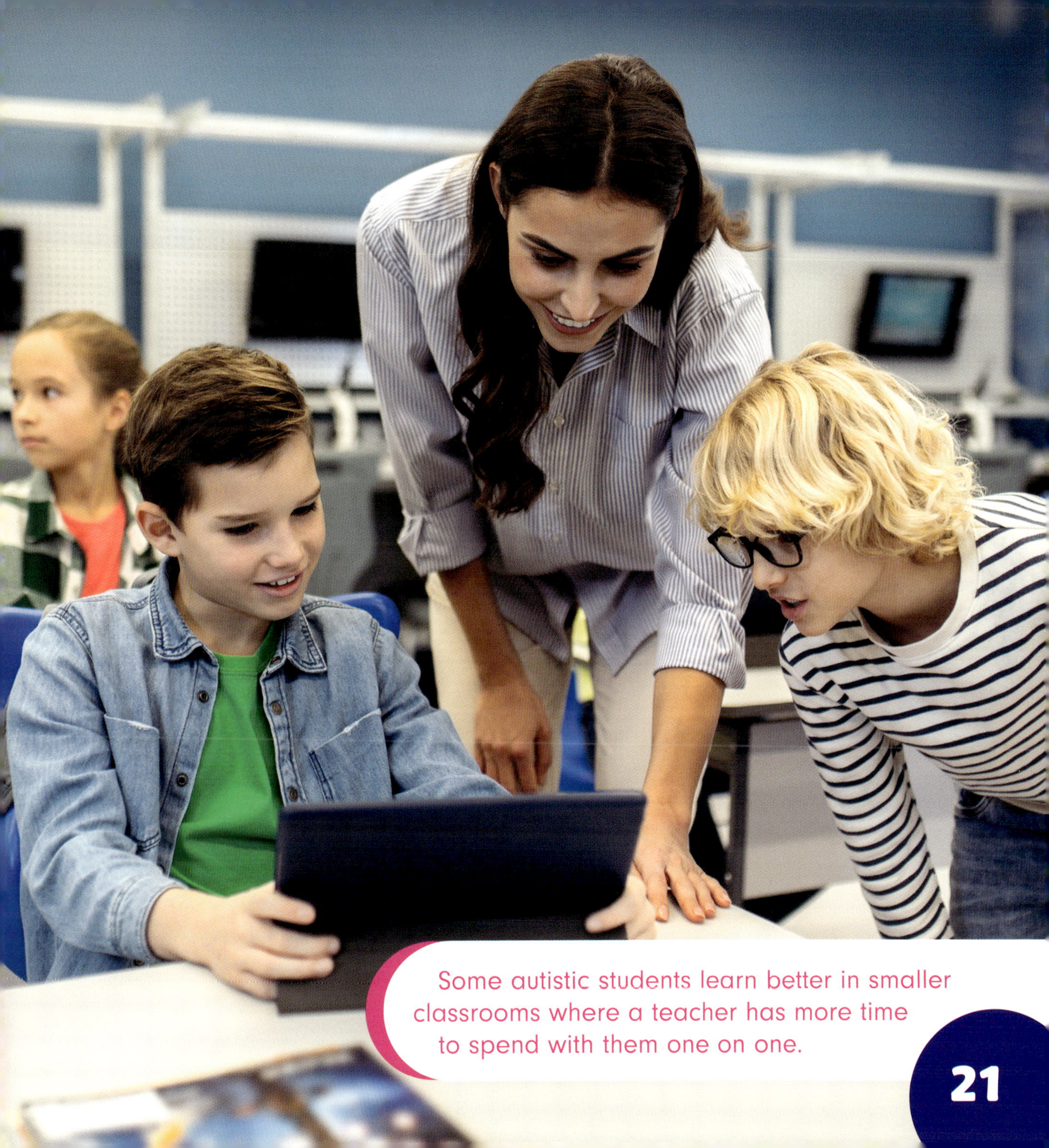

Some autistic students learn better in smaller classrooms where a teacher has more time to spend with them one on one.

Glossary

affect: To act on or change something.

anxious: Having a feeling of unease or worry.

communication: The use of words, sounds, signs, or behaviors to convey ideas, thoughts, and feelings.

counselor: A person who gives advice or help.

diagnose: To identify a disease or issue by its signs and symptoms.

future: Something that has yet to be.

mental: Having to do with the mind.

syndrome: An illness, disorder, or condition concerning the body or mind.

therapist: A type of health care worker who specializes in a certain treatment.

treatment: A method for helping someone who is ill or has a medical condition

For More Information

Books

Rusick, Jessica. *Understanding Autism*. Minneapolis, MN: ABDO Publishing Company, 2021.

Verdick, Elizabeth, and Elizabeth Reeve. *The Survival Guide for Kids with Autism Spectrum Disorder (And Their Parents)*. Minneapolis, MN: Free Spirit Publishing, 2021.

Websites

Britannica Kids
www.kids.britannica.com/kids/article/autism/544837
Learn more about autism.

Kids Health
kidshealth.org/en/kids/autism.html
Read helpful information about living with autism.

Index